BEAUTY:

WHAT IT IS, AND HOW

TO RETAIN IT.

BY A LADY.

"Whatever you have, have beauty."
SYDNEY SMITH.

PREFACE.

THE great success of " How to Dress on £15 a Year," has induced the Publishers to issue this little companion volume, on a subject equally interesting and important, trusting that it may find equal favour with English ladies.

London, Sept., 1873.

First published in 1873 by Frederick Warne & Co, London

This edition published in 2012 by
The British Library
96 Euston Road
London NW1 2DB

British Library Cataloguing in Publication Data
A catalogue record for this publication is available from
The British Library

ISBN 978 0 7123 5885 9

Printed in Hong Kong by Great Wall Printing Co. Ltd

BEAUTY.

PRELIMINARY CHAPTER.

Beauty a great power—Former objections to discussion of the
    subject—Changes of opinion—Greek value for beauty—
    Taste for beauty, and how formed—Passages from the ancient
    and modern poets—Necessity of a just sense of the beautiful.

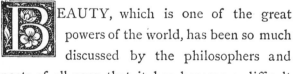EAUTY, which is one of the great
powers of the world, has been so much
discussed by the philosophers and
poets of all ages, that it has become a difficult
subject to write about in these latter ages.   Yet,
before beginning the more practical portion of
this little book, we are tempted to say a few

words on the subject, as some excuse for calling attention to the matter at all.

With certain people it was at one time considered a sinful vanity to think about personal beauty. The body was to be treated by all wise people with contemptuous indifference. The subject of good looks was to be eschewed in the presence of children; and the most lovely young girl was never permitted to become aware of her personal perfections (so far as her guardians could prevent it) till she learned them suddenly by her success in society.

This was surely a greater trial to her moral nature than if she had from infancy heard that God had bestowed a great and precious gift on her, which she must learn to use aright, and of which she had no just reason to be proud.

We have changed all this; muscular Christianity restored to the human frame that due regard which *all* men owe to it; and the new and more artistic sense of beauty which undoubtedly sprang from the great Exhibition of 1851, has rendered people more inclined to discuss beauty as an important and valuable gift, which, like all other good gifts of Heaven, requires and deserves our careful attention.

The wise Greeks ever estimated it at its just value. Aristotle has told us that a graceful person is a more powerful recommendation than the best letter that can be written in one's favour; Socrates called it "a short-lived tyranny," thus, at least, acknowledging its power; Theophrastus termed it "a silent fraud," meaning that it can impose on us without the aid of language; Carneades calls it "royalty without force," *i.e.*, a sway which requires no effort to enforce it.

Knowing and feeling this, they cultivated personal beauty, till they became the first in form as in intellect of the human race—a connection inevitable, by-the-bye, when the former is really perfect; for without the inner soul of beauty there is no external perfection.

The idea of beauty differed then, however, as it does now, amongst various nations, each selecting that type most characteristic of its nationality. The stately aquiline-featured Roman women were as beautiful in Roman eyes as if they had possessed the delicate brow and straight nose of the Greeks; and the dusky splendour of the Ethiop Queen was doubtless thought superior to both by her countrymen. This preference for a familiar cast of features and complexion, is doubtless a blessing to the nations, but has led to strange notions of beauty.

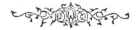

The taste for beauty requires cultivation, and in Europe, has probably been preserved through the changes of time and fashion, by the poets, even more than by the painters.

Here is a very vivid picture of Greek beauty, translated by Moore:

> Best of painters, come portray
> The lovely maid that's far away—
> Far away, my soul, thou art,
> But I've thy beauties all by heart.
> Paint her jetty ringlets straying,
> Silky twine in tendrils playing;
> And if painting hath the skill

To make the spicy balm distil,
Let every little lock exhale
A sigh of perfume on the gale.
Where her tresses' curly flow,
Darkles o'er the brow of snow,
Let her forehead beam to light,
Burnished as the ivory bright ;
Let her eyebrows sweetly rise
In jetty arches o'er her eyes :
Gently in a crescent gliding—
Just commingling—just dividing.
But hast thou any sparkles warm,
The lightning of her eyes to form ?
Let them effuse the azure ray
With which Minerva's glances play.

*   *   *   *   *

O'er her nose and cheek be shed
Flushing white and mellow red—
Gradual tints, as when there glows
In snowy milk the bashful rose.

*   *   *   *   *

Paint where the ruby cell uncloses :
Persuasion sleeping upon roses ;
*   *   *   The velvet chin,
Whose dimple shades a love within.

A very perfect picture of external beauty this, yet lacking a something, to be supplied by the poets of another and a better civilization.

"The Romans," says Longepièrre, "were so convinced of the power of beauty, that they used a word implying strength in the place of the epithet 'beautiful.' See Plautus's 'Bacchi,' Act II., Scene 2." They admired auburn or golden hair, and dyed their dark locks of that colour. The taste lingered long in Italy, and in the sixteenth century, golden locks were immortalized by the great Italian painters.

The poets of Christendom have idealized a higher order of beauty — that in which moral and intellectual loveliness inform and exalt mere matter.

Compare Spenser's Una with the Greek beauty, and the difference will be at once perceptible :

> From her fair head her fillet she undight,
>   And laid her stole aside ; her *angel's face*
> As the great eye of heaven shined bright,
>   And made a sunshine in that shady place—
> Did never mortal eye behold such heavenly grace.

Or read the description of Spenser's bride :

> Her long loose yellow locks, like golden wire,
>   Sprinkled with pearl and pearling flowers atween,
> Do like a golden mantle her attire,
>   And being crownèd with a garland green,
>   Seem like some maiden queen.

Her *modest eyes*, abashèd to behold
  So many gazers as on her do stare,
  Upon the lowly ground affixèd are ;
Ne dare lift up her countenance too bold,
  But blush to hear her praises sung so loud.

*   *   *   *   *   *

Tell me, ye merchants' daughters, did ye see
  So fair a creature in your town before ?—
So sweet, so lovely, and so mild as she,
  Adorned with Beauty's grace and Virtue's store?
Her goodly eyes like sapphires shining bright ;
    Her forehead ivory white ;
Her cheeks like apples which the sun hath rudded ;
Her lips like cherries . . . . .

But if ye saw that which no eye can see—
  The inward beauty of her lively sprite,
Garnished with heavenly gifts of high degree—
  Much more then would you wonder at the sight !
There dwells sweet Love and constant Chastity,
  Unspotted Faith and comely Womanhood,
Regard of honour and mild modesty ;
  There Virtue reigns as queen in regal throne,
    And giveth laws alone.

Drayton, a poet of the same period, gives us
this charming picture of a woman's hand :

  So white, so soft, so delicate, so sleek—
    As she had worn a lily for a glove !

Shakspeare's women impress us with their
beauty without details. We see Imogen as the

"fresh lily" he calls her; Desdemona as "one entire and perfect chrysolite;" Perdita's loveliness, as "the prettiest Lowland lass that treads the greensward," is present to us; and Juliet's beauty, which "teaches the torches to burn bright," steals into our mind with a glow of southern loveliness. Milton's Eve is a wonderful picture of stately beauty :

> Grace was in all her steps, heaven in her eyes—
> In every gesture dignity and love.

Here, too, is a far loftier ideal than the Greek.

Our modern poets, too, have given us charming ideas of beauty. Byron's description of Zuleika is, perhaps, one of the finest, and is well known.

Keats gives us a picture of Diana, not, we think, inferior to the Greek sketch of beauty :

> Speak, stubborn earth, and tell me where, O where
> Hast thou a symbol of her golden hair?
> Not *oat-sheaves drooping in the western sun ;*
> *　　*　　*　　*　　Yet she had,
> Indeed, locks bright enough to make me mad—
> And they were gordianed up and braided,
> Leaving, in naked comeliness, unshaded
> Her pearl-round ears, white neck, and orbéd brow :
> The which were blended in I know not how

With such a paradise of lips and eyes,
Blush-tinted cheeks, half-smiles, and faintest sighs,
That when I think thereon, my spirit clings
And plays about its fancy, till the stings
Of human neighbourhood envenom all.
*   *   *   Ah! see her hovering feet,
More bluely veined, more soft, more whitely sweet,
Than those of sea-born Venus when she rose
From out her cradle shell.

Then we have the charming picture of Nourmahal, in Moore, which should never be omitted
when we talk of the poets' ideal of beauty:

There's a beauty for ever unchangingly bright,
Like the long sunny lapse of a summer day's light;
Shining on, shining on, by no shadow made tender,
Till Love falls asleep in its sameness of splendour.
This was not the beauty—oh! nothing like this
That to young Nourmahal gave such magic of bliss;
But that loveliness ever in motion, which plays
Like the light upon autumn's soft shadowy days—
Now here, and now there, giving warmth as it flies
From the lips to the cheek, from the cheek to the eyes.

It is upon these word-pictures that we have
formed our ideas of beauty, and gathered fair
visions of female loveliness, whose presence
enlivens and adorns the world of which it is one
of the joys and blessings.

The painters and sculptors, too, have helped form our ideal, and their dicta are taken into account in the following chapters.

A just sense of the beautiful, a rational love of it, an innocent desire to cultivate and preserve this good gift of God, cannot do otherwise than benefit those whose dowry it is from Heaven; and who have no right to despise or neglect it; or to tamper with and destroy it by absurd artifices, which would meet with the unqualified contempt they deserve if women had better knowledge on the subject—a knowledge which it is the aim of this little work to give.

CHAPTER II.

BEAUTY OF FORM.

English beauty—What we owe to it—Beauty in the present day
a national possession—Duty of preserving good looks—The
figure—Shoulders—Waist—Feet—Walk—Methods of improving the figure and walk—Exercise and diet.

NGLAND has been justly styled the
land of beauty, and to this good gift
of God she has been infinitely indebted; for it was to the beauty of Saxon children that she owes her Christianity. "Not Angles,
but angels!" cried St. Gregory, as he gazed on
the golden-haired Anglo-Saxons, in the slave-
market of Rome. And assuredly up to the present day this good gift has not failed us. No
race of men equal the stalwart sons of Britain,

no maidens are so fair ; in no country is beauty more lasting.

An ugly English girl is an anomaly. With the unrivalled British complexion, it is rare for a maiden to fail of possessing what our neighbours call *la beauté du diable.* But of all women in Europe, English women do least to improve or preserve their beauty. They follow fashion, however absurd, in a blind aimless way, being content to do as every one else does, and having but very hazy notions of what true beauty is. They will pinch in their feet and waists, paint their faces, dye their hair ; but as to any real knowledge of *how really* to improve the precious gift committed to their trust, they are ignorant.

The perception of beauty we are well aware is not a distinct faculty : it is a matter of opinion and feeling, controlled and directed by national prejudices, early impressions, education, and a cultivated and refined taste.

> Who hath not proved how feebly words essay
> To fix one spark of Beauty's heavenly ray ?

In actual life, women who possess what is called "charm" have generally been the beauties of their period—not those who are the nearest embodiment of the sculptor's ideal. It is more than probable that Cleopatra's fascination lay rather in her "strong toil of grace" and her "infinite variety" than in her Ethiopian features and dark complexion; and the portraits of Mary of Scotland, Joanna of Naples, and Venetia Digby do not strike us as possessing anything extraordinary in point of features. These women charmed people, and were justly declared to be beautiful.

Nevertheless, there is a certain artistic rule of personal beauty grown out of the taste of painters and poets, which may guide us to that which is as near an approach to beauty as mere form can be; always premising that the indefinable charm of beauty will not be found in the perfection of form or feature without the informing mind which Plato has declared to be alone beautiful.

> The light of love, the purity of grace,
> The mind, the music breathing from her face;
> The heart whose softness harmonized the whole,

as Byron exquisitely describes his "Zuleika."

But though we may fully acknowledge Plato's doctrine, that in perceiving beauty, the mind only contemplates the shadow of its own affections, still a near external approach to those forms which taste has definitely settled as beautiful, is desirable. We believe few of our readers are aware in what a high degree this approach may be facilitated by pains and attention. All the gifts entrusted to us by nature demand our best care—and, to woman especially, beauty is a gift of vast moment, for in it lies much of her power for good or evil.

It is one of her minor morals to look as well she can; for beauty enlisted on the side of goodness, is one of its most potent arms against evil.

But let us return to the practical view of the subject, which is the design of our little volume.

We will begin with the FIGURE, which is really of more importance than the face, because it belongs to that "strong toil of grace" of which we have already spoken.

"The beauty of the female figure," says Leigh Hunt, "consists in being gently serpentine." Stiffness is utterly ungraceful.

The movements of an unconscious child are the perfection of grace; they are easy, unstudied, natural.

The THROAT should be round, full, and pillar-like. Chaucer describing—it is believed—the beautiful Blanche of Lancaster, says,

> Her throte, as I have now memoire,
> Seemed as a *round tower* of yvoire (ivory),
> Of *good greteness* and not too grete.

The WAIST should be *twice* the size of this "tower of ivory," *not*, as fashion has too often made it, nearly the same size.

The SHOULDERS should be falling, and not too broad (very broad shoulders being a masculine beauty); but they had better be broad than too narrow, as any contraction across the chest gives a mean and pinched look to the person. The figure should be easy; too small a waist is an actual deformity, and we may remind young ladies who labour under the delusion of thinking that a waist of eighteen inches is lovely, that that of the Venus de' Medici, the acknowledged type of female beauty, measures twenty-seven inches.

When these deformed waists are made by tight lacing, they not only mar the beauty of the figure, but injure that of the face, by giving a red tip to the nose. In fact, tight ligatures anywhere about the person are apt, by impeding the circulation, to paint the nose, by no means charmingly, and to thicken the ankles; not to speak of the injury to the health, and through that to the general complexion.

The HIPS should be high in a woman, and wide; the FEET small, but in due proportion to the height of the figure. A high instep is beautiful, and a hollowing in the sole is considered by the Arabs a mark of high birth.

Nevertheless, the foot should not be made so small—by means of tight boots—as to mar the perfect gracefulness of the walk.

Ariosto describes a beautiful foot as "*breve, asciutto, e ritondetto*," that is, "short, neat, and a little rounded," *i.e.*, not thin. The Chinese have made a deformity of a beauty by exaggerating it, and one shudders at all their women underwent in ancient times to attain this horrible fashionable disfigurement. But we have been told by the daughter of a Chinese lady, that they have greatly changed in this respect, and (like Europeans) now feign the imaginary grace. The foot is made to appear very short, by wearing immensely high heels, which show the toe on its point, and by raising the foot nearly perpendicularly, diminish its apparent length as much as they desire it to be diminished, and produce the same crippled stumbling walk.

The present fashion of our women of wearing the high heels nearly in the centre of the sole, produces in a degree the same effect.

The doctors object to these high heels as injurious in the extreme.*

We do not deny that moderately high heels (in their right place) have a certain smartness, when they do not injure the walk, the gracefulness of which is most important.

——Pedes vestis defluxit ad imos
Et vera incessu patuit Dea——

* The very high heels recently worn have produced a new and serious complaint of the feet, requiring, to cure it, a painful operation.

says Virgil—that is, Venus wore a long train, and was known *by her graceful walk* to be a goddess.

> In length of train descends her sweeping gown,
> And by her graceful walk the queen of love is known.
> DRYDEN.

We have long acknowledged the grace and dignity given by length of train; it is to be desired that the graceful walk were more sought after by our women. To attain it, the movement must be made from the hip; it will not then shake the garments; the waist being still, except from that gentle, willowy, swaying motion which accompanies the movements of the most graceful figures.

One of the best modes of attaining a walk from the hip, is to practise walking with something poised on the head. The graceful Hindoo girl can bear a pitcher on her head, unsupported by the hand, simply because she moves from the hip, instead of from the waist—a mode of walking which the necessity of pitcher-carrying probably originally induced.

Before leaving this subject, we would urge on

our lady readers the benefit to be derived (both to health and form) from simple arm exercises.

If, every night before they slept, they went through two, which we will indicate, contracted chests and high shoulders might be avoided.

Exercise I.—Stand with the heels together and the feet turned out slightly. The knees should be tightened so as to be effaced, and the weight of the body should be thrown on the front part of the foot, not on the heels. Then raise the hands side by side, finger-tips upwards, in the middle of the chest. Pull them with a jerk back to the shoulders, and then let the arms fall straight down.

Exercise II.—Stand in the same position. Put the tips of the fingers to the shoulders; the elbows against the sides. Drop the arms strongly, having the palms of the hands turned outwards.

This exercise pulls down the shoulders, as the other expands the chest. These simple gymnastics will be found quite sufficient for young ladies content to be only graceful. They will suffice for forming and preserving the figure.

People who sit much and are in the habit of bending over sedentary employments, lose the elastic grace peculiar to those who walk or ride regularly.

Too great stoutness or thinness is to be avoided : the former by vigorous exercise and a careful diet ; eschewing great quantities of the flesh-forming or fat-creating foods. Animal food is less fattening than bread, vegetables, and puddings ; beer and porter are to be avoided by too fat people, and claret substituted in their place.

But starving for the figure is a folly, which brings its punishment in a leaden complexion and dull eyes. Plumpness, be it remembered, is beautiful ; great thinness, or, as it is called, *scragginess,* is ugly ; and one thing is certain— the compression of the figure, even *if* too much inclined to *embonpoint,* is a mistake. A pinched-in waist will only give a too great exuberance of flesh above and below it, and thus reveal itself as false.

Corsets have been the bane of English figures.

The models for sculptors and painters in Italy are *never* allowed to wear corsets, for fear of spoiling the figure. This fact speaks volumes in explanation of the defects of English shapes. Happily fashion has introduced the short French corset, and our women have escaped, if they please, from the iron cages in which their grand-mothers lived—the high, long, stiff "stays" which made *them* stiff, straight, and unshapely, and precluded every shadow of grace.

If the future generation were never to wear corsets at all, we might hope for a general im-provement in the race, both male and female, but this at present seems a consummation only to be hoped for.

But hope it we shall! for much has been done in the way of enlightening our women on this matter—and "scragginess" is no longer esteemed lovely. Sylphs have given way to "fine animals," and the exchange is for the better as far as both health and beauty go.

For the too thin ladies we would recommend a generous diet and porter—which fattens best,

we believe; also suet puddings and butter in
abundance; and the cultivation of cheerfulness
and good nature.

Their defects are of an easier nature to redeem by art, than those of too ponderous
beauties, and a supple grace will atone for
even meagreness.

We are not, remember, disparaging a slight
rounded figure, or advocating an Eastern stand-
ard of beauty by weight, but speaking of figures
in which thinness has degenerated into gauntness.

We have spoken much of grace—What is it?
Such an indescribable thing, that we know
not well how to write on it with any chance of
giving a good idea of it to the naturally ungraceful. Negatives may, however, help us. It
is not graceful to walk with the defiant stump
peculiar to the "fast" girl, who, though she
may be a very "good fellow," loses a great
portion of her "toil of grace" when she
abandons

> Fear and niceness,
> The handmaids of all women, or more truly,
> Woman its pretty self.—SHAKSPEARE.

Nor is it graceful to square the elbows as in driving a pair of horses, or to move with sharp jerky movements. To be graceful a woman should not be habitually hurried and in a fuss; she should take time to move, and care (at first) in making all movements quietly. By degrees it will become habitual to be graceful.

But the greatest foe of grace is self-consciousness. This alone will spoil both it and beauty. Byron's heroine "who never thought about herself at all," was doubtless as graceful as Cleopatra. A woman who puts her individual self aside altogether, cannot fail of attaining a certain sort of grace, because she will be perfectly at her ease.

Frenchwomen are more graceful than Englishwomen, because they are less self-conscious. A Frenchwoman unexpectedly brought into the presence of strangers, in an old or otherwise unfitting dress, will directly forget it, in entertaining her guests, and by the charm of her own ease will make her bad dress pass unobserved. An Englishwoman is instantly painfully conscious of every defect of toilette, and becomes awkward because she cannot forget *herself*.

This half-vain half-modest self-consciousness in former days caused affectation; in the present day it has a less baneful effect, but it produces awkwardness and a blunt ungraceful manner.

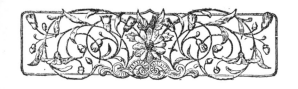

CHAPTER III.

FORM AND COLOUR.

The beauty of the arm—Outline—Colour—Movements—The
hand—Shape—Colour—Nails—To whiten the hands—
Red hands—Cause and cure—Expression of the hand—
Manipulations—Rings.

THE ARM should have a round and flowing outline, with no sharpness of the elbows: it should taper gently down to a small wrist. Thin arms are ugly, and require graceful movements to make us forget their sharpness. A white arm is beautiful, but a dark-complexioned arm may be more beautiful if it is better shaped, form being the chief loveliness of the arm.

The movements of the arm give either awkwardness or grace to the person. They should never be sharp or angular, but rounded, without affectation. Keeping the elbows away from the sides in a sharp angle is very ungraceful; and the habit (unknown to our grandmothers) of crossing the arms on the chest when sitting, *à la* Napoleon's pictures, or putting the hands in the jacket pockets, alike detract from feminine grace.

The HAND should be long and delicate, yet plump, with taper fingers, the tips of which, when the hand rests on its palm, should turn back a little. There is scarcely any charm of beauty which surpasses that of a beautiful hand. Whiteness is essential to it, but the finger-nails ought to have a rosy tinge, and also the palm of the hand.

Our readers will perceive at once that the beauty of a well-formed hand will depend for the loveliness of complexion on the circulation. Imperfect circulation gives the blue tinge we see in some hands in winter, or the red look, which is equally objectionable.

Perfect health, necessary for the complexion,

is of course essential to the hand. A sickly-looking hand, however white, may move tenderness and pity, but is not beautiful.

The NAILS will often mar or make the beauty of a hand. They should be kept perfectly clean. Every morning, after washing the hands, the skin which grows up from the bottom and round the side of the nail should be pressed back with the towel or with a little ivory instrument sold for the purpose ; but the nail must never be scraped, as scraping produces wrinkles on it —those lines down the nail that mar its beauty.

Before cutting them, the nails should be held in very warm water, to make them soft and flexible, then they should be cut in the form of a half moon for the hands, and square (nearly) for the feet.

To keep or render the hands white, they should occasionally (after a good washing with glycerine soap) be rubbed with lemon-juice and water.

Red hands are caused by want of proper circulation, and are peculiar to the debateable age between youth and womanhood. Constant exercise, electricity, and warm gloves, and keeping the wrist covered are the best means of restoring their colour. Whenever the hands are inclined to become red, warm milk and water should be used to them at night before going to bed.

The hands should never be suffered to remain long soiled with anything that will stain them. After gardening, drawing in chalk, &c., they should be washed *at once* in soft warm water, and, if stained, pumice-stone should be used. But unless there is some reason for it, it is better not to wash the hands very often. They should be dried with a soft towel and powdered with violet powder.

In winter the hands should be washed with oatmeal and warm soft water to prevent chapping ; or, if chapped, camphor ball and glycerine should be rubbed on at night.

Chilblains on the hands are to be carefully guarded against, as they always leave disfiguring protuberances on the finger-joints. Very young girls, or persons who take little exercise, are subject to them from want of circulation,

They must be most carefully guarded against, by never holding very cold hands to the fire to warm; and next, by never omitting daily exercise.

The hands should be well dried and strongly rubbed after washing, and covered from the out-door cold. Electricity received into the system prevents chilblains.

When they appear, the following wash is recommended for them:

Chilblain Wash.—Two ounces of sal ammoniac to be placed in one quart of *rain*-water; put it on the fire and let it boil till the sal ammoniac is dissolved.

N.B.—It must be rain-water, and not applied near the fire, but rubbed on the chilblains two or three times a day.

Should the chilblain break, it may be dressed twice daily with a plaster made of the following ointment :—One ounce of hog's lard, one ounce of bees'wax, and half an ounce of oil of turpentine; melt these and mix them thoroughly, spread on leather, and apply immediately.

Sunburn ought not to exist on the hands, as even when gardening they may be kept covered with old gloves ; but if the hands chance to get browned, lemon-juice should be used to remove the tan.

For freckles (which are a great blemish on the hands and arms, and give a common look) make and apply the following mixture :— Lemon-juice, one ounce ; powdered borax, one quarter of a drachm ; sugar, half a drachm. Keep it in a glass bottle for a few days, and apply occasionally.

Pumice-stone will remove stains of fruit and ink. Warts may be removed by tying a piece of raw beef, soaked for twenty-four hours previously in vinegar, over them. In a week, if it is worn constantly ; and, in a fortnight, if it is worn only at night, the wart will disappear and leave no scar on the flesh. Warts from the face may be removed in the same way, by fastening the vinegar-soaked meat on by strips of sticking plaster.

Old gloves with the tips cut off are serviceable

in preserving the hands white, and do not mar
their usefulness.

The hand should look able to move swiftly
and skilfully. There is much expression in it.
A lymphatic lazy hand is easily distinguished
from the hand of the artist or musician. Good
manipulations impart character and grace to it.

Rings, when elegant, embellish the hand, and
are perhaps the most graceful ornament of the
young, but *too many* of them cripple and disfigure
the fingers.

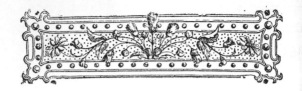

CHAPTER IV.

THE HEAD AND HAIR.

Shape of the head—Breadth—Depth—Pose on the shoulders—
Hair—Colours—Quantity—Grey hair—Dyeing and its
effects—Strengthening the hair—Modes of dressing it.

THE shape of the HEAD is beautiful in
proportion as it inclines from round
into oval. Its size should be an eighth
part of the height of the whole figure. The larger
the facial angle the more intellectual the head is
supposed to be.

The facial angle is an angle which results from
union of two lines, one of which touches the fore
head, the other of which, drawn from the orifice of
the ear, meets the former line at the extremity of

the front teeth. In the Greek statues it is an angle of 90°.

The chief breadth of the head should be at the temples and over the ears. It should be gracefully poised on the body.

<blockquote>Beauty draws us with a single hair,</blockquote>

is scarcely a poetical exaggeration; and the fashion of dressing and adorning the HAIR has always been important—even in King Solomon's days, whose boy pages, we are told by Josephus, wore gold-dust powdered on their jetty locks!

Hair should be abundant, soft, long, and fine. Of late years the favourite hue of the ancients and of the poets of the fifteenth century, golden or auburn, has resumed its former sway (with the revival of that sense of colour so long dormant amongst us); and every shade of red has flaunted itself before us, till the dark-haired beauties have been tempted to imitate it by dyes, to the great detriment of their appearance, as the harmony between the colour of the down on the cheek and the hair is thus destroyed, and also the gloss and life of the hair. No dye can give the

Gold upon a crown of jet,

of which Ben Jonson sang.

Black and rich brown hair—the one with the
purple light of a raven's wing on it, the other
burnished as with gold, will always hold their
own against light or red hair, and are beautiful,
whatever may be the fashion. They are remarkable also for possessing a faint perfume
occasionally, as if scented, and are always in this
way pleasanter than fair hair.

We may be sure, whatever colour the hair
may be, that it is the one precisely best suited
to the complexion and eyes with which we
find it.

Nature is a cunning painter, and well under-
stands the harmony of colouring. When we
dye, we disfigure both our hair and our complexion.

Dyeing the hair, by-the-bye, has been practised
in nearly all ages. In the sixteenth century the
Venetian ladies had a singular fashion of dyeing
it in locks of various colours, all worn at the same
time, and which, floating over their shoulders,

from their crownless hats, must have had a very strange appearance. It was at this time that their *chopines*, the precursors of our ladies' high-heeled boots, rendered them unable to walk without assistance.*

The hair thus dyed must have had an unpleasant effect on the complexion, for, as we have said, there is on the skin a soft down—occasionally visible on lovely brunette skins—which would be a horrid contrast to the hair of many colours.

This down changes with the hair, and becomes whiter as the hair silvers. It is this which gives such a hard, even fierce, look to the countenance when false black hair or dyed black hair is substituted for grey.

When dye is used (but it is *always* a mistake, and often a dangerous one) it should be light in

---

* A Venetian beauty, wearing the rim only of a broad hat, her hair of many hues streaming from the place where "the crown ought to be," and only able to walk upon her stilt-like *chopines* by leaning on two attendants, must have been a very picture of the utter foolishness to which fashion may descend.

colour, to prevent this harsh contrast with the skin. But there is not such a thing as an innoxious dye for the hair, if we except the two vegetable ones—walnut-juice, and mullein and genista. The former dyes the hair, but also blackens and stains the skin, which shows the stain at the partings. Mullein and genista are the best. The receipt is half an ounce of the flowers of mullein and half an ounce of genista, stewed in water till the liquor is quite black. To be applied daily with a sponge, when the result will be achieved. We are indebted for this receipt to some amusing articles in "Land and Water" on this subject. For premature grey hair, this vegetable dye has been found useful.

Grey hair, the glory of old age, is apt in the present day to arrive before befitting years, and then an innocuous dye is not so objectionable.

We would warn our fair readers against pulling out grey hairs. It is quite possible that improved health may restore their colour—we have seen an instance of this in our own family; and if not, the soft grey hair which has never been uprooted (or broken off under the delusion of uprooting it) will always lie hidden amongst the hair; while the grey hairs which grow again after being pulled out, are stiff, short, and have a habit of standing erect! Never pull out a grey hair.

But prevention is better than cure. How are ladies to preserve the colour and abundance of their tresses? We believe that the best and most important rule for so doing, is to keep the head cool and clean. But the former is nearly an impossibility in these days of frizettes and false hair. One thing, however, is certain. If our ladies would preserve their own abundant tresses for another (and probably widely different) fashion, they must get the head cool during the night and before dressing the hair the next morning. To effect this, the hair must be taken down and well brushed at night with a soft brush, parting it about, to cool and clean it; and then it should be plaited and suffered to hang about the shoulders all night. In the morning the roots should be well washed with rose-water, or *cold soft (or rain) water*, if possible—the latter is best. Then it must be dried, before it is dressed, by rubbing gently and shaking out, or brushing with a soft brush.

This treatment will remove scurf, which is, we believe, one of the causes of premature grey hair, and which undoubtedly weakens the roots of the hair, and prevents it from growing, besides being horribly unsightly. When, after washing carefully, the scurf is found nearly as bad as ever, a lotion must be used, of one ounce of glycerine in eight ounces of rose-water; this will render the skin soft and clean, and improve the hair. Even in cases of skin disease in the head, this lotion will be found efficacious.

Brushing should be performed carefully. Where it is possible the hair should be brushed by another person; but as all our readers cannot have ladies' maids, we advise them to divide the hair at the back of the head and brush it from each side gently. If entangled, it should be freed from knots by beginning a little way up from the ends of the hair and gradually brushing from above, care being taken not to break the hair, which should be brushed for twenty minutes night and morning.

The abundant false hair used in the present day, and which may be tolerated because it is openly worn and makes no attempt at deception —"what she spends or has spent on her hair" being frankly discussed by our maidens amongst themselves—requires great care and attention on the part of the owner or her maid to keep clean and fresh.

Large skeins of hair, which can be cleaned and dressed often, are greatly to be preferred to the chignons made up in rolls, &c., &c., originally sold. The niceness and cleanliness of these coils are absolutely essential to their adding beauty to the wearer, as in no case is the proverb "Cleanliness is next to goodliness," (*i.e.* beauty,) more true than in all matters respecting the hair—dirty false or natural hair being equally detestable.

But, as we have said before, fashions change; false hair may go out of fashion in a few years' time, and *then* the ladies who have preserved their own hair in any quantity will have cause to rejoice.　Now everybody knows how prone the hair is to fall off, especially under its modern assimilation with borrowed tresses.

When it gets thin and meagre, what is best to be done to renew its growth?

The ends should be well cut, *frequently*, and a stimulating lotion used to help the hair-follicle to secretion.　Stimulants and cutting are the only remedy.

The best stimulating washes we know are made thus:—One ounce of spirit of turpentine, one ounce of trotter oil, thirty drops of acetic solution of cantharides.

Another good wash to make the hair grow is: Camphor, one drachm; borax, one ditto; spirits of wine, two teaspoonfuls; tincture of cantharides, two teaspoonfuls; rosemary oil, four drops; rosewater, half a pint.　Dissolve the camphor and borax in the spirit, add the oil, and lastly shake it up gradually with the rose-water.

Mr. Erasmus Wilson gives the following receipt for strengthening the hair and preventing its falling off:—Vinegar of cantharides, half an ounce;

eau de Cologne, one ounce; rose-water, one ounce. The scalp should be brushed briskly until it becomes red, and the lotion should then be applied to the roots of the hair twice a day.

Of ordinary washes there are many useful ones; one of the very nicest is made of box and rosemary-leaves, each one handful, boiled in a quart of water till it becomes a pint. Strain, and when cold add half a gill of rum. Pour into bottles and cork them down. This wash will keep for a long time, and is remarkably clean and nice to use.

Glycerine, half an ounce; spirit of rosemary, half an ounce; water, five ounces; to be well mixed and shaken; to be used daily—is also to be recommended.

Some little time back there appeared three or four brief articles in "Land and Water," called "Secrets of Beauty." The writer recommends a decoction of strong green tea, stewed till it is nearly the colour of coffee, as a marvellous wash for the hair, promoting its growth and improving it generally. Our only doubt about this is its power of dyeing, which is great. We have often tinted our drawing-paper with a decoction of green tea, and it is used also for washing black lace, the colour of which it restores. Would it give a (temporary) green tinge to the hair? We cannot answer this question, as we have not tried the prescription.

With regard to the mode of wearing the hair, so much depends on fashion, that no directions can be given.

It is a fact that whatever is fashionable becomes pleasing to the eye—probably from association. But in the present day individual taste is permitted to modify and adapt fashion in a great degree, and it is in this that good taste is displayed. The present mode has a certain style about it, and we think the hair rolled off the forehead and worn high, is peculiarly becoming to short round faces and low foreheads.

The mode of wearing the hair should be studied by each individual, and the fashion modified to that which is most becoming to the wearer.

We shall conclude these remarks on the hair with some receipts for pomade, &c., &c.

French Pomatum.—Lard, four ounces; honey, four ounces; the best olive oil, two ounces. Melt the above together, and let it stand till cold, when the honey will sink to the bottom; then melt it once again without the honey. Scent it with a quarter of an ounce of essence of bitter almonds, put in with the liquid after the second melting, essence of jessamine, or otto of roses.

Pomade for the Hair.—Beef marrow, four ounces; lard, two ounces; salad oil, three table-spoonfuls; some good scent. Clarify the beef marrow, and let it stand until cold. Clarify the lard, and when cold beat it to a cream and add it to the marrow. Put both into a saucepan, and let it boil until well mixed, stirring it constantly. Then add the oil and any scent you prefer. Pour it into pots or glass bottles, and it will be fit for use.

Soft Pomatum.—Take two pounds of hog's lard, boil and skim it well, put into it a small quantity of hair powder. When it is cool scent it with essence of lemon and bergamot.

Hair-Curling Fluid.—The only curling fluid

of any service is a weak solution of isinglass, which will hold the curl in the position in which it is placed, if care is taken that it follows the direction in which the hair naturally falls.

One of the fluids in use is made by dissolving a small portion of bees'wax in an ounce of olive oil, and adding scent according to taste.

Bandoline.—1. Simmer an ounce of quince-seed in a quart of water for forty minutes; strain, cool, add a few drops of scent, and bottle, corking tightly.

2. Take of gum tragacanth one and a half drachm; water, half a pint; rectified spirits mixed with an equal quantity of water, three ounces; and a little scent. Let the mixture stand for a day or two, then strain.

3. It may be made of Iceland moss, a quarter of an ounce boiled in a quart of water, and a little rectified spirit added, so that it may keep.

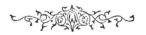

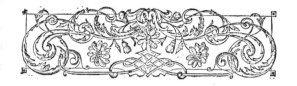

CHAPTER V.

THE UPPER PART OF THE FACE.

The Forehead—Eyes—Eyelids—Eyebrows.

THE FOREHEAD should be straight, compact, and not too high.

"A forehead," says Junius, "should be smooth, even, white, delicate, short, and of an open and cheerful character." "*Di terso avorio era la fronte lieta*," says Ariosto ("Of terse ivory was the joyous brow"); a brow, that is, smooth and not disfigured by frowns, which speedily leave their indelible marks on it. Care should be taken in youth, not to make straight long lines on the forehead by the habit of lifting the eyebrows—a senseless trick, which gives the countenance quite early an appearance of age. The forehead will occasionally grow rough from exposure in boats or on horseback. It should then be lightly brushed over with some fine olive oil, but cold cream and every animal grease should *never* be applied to the human skin.

For a low forehead the hair should be worn rolled up off it. When it grows low in front and high at the sides, the present fashion will be found very becoming, as the height on the temples will show. Care should be taken not needlessly to tan the forehead.

A very high round forehead requires the hair to be worn lower over it than a low broad one.

The EYES are, perhaps, the greatest personal beauty. The soul looks out of them. All colours may be beautiful. Black eyes are supposed to be most intellectual; blue eyes the most soft and tender; grey eyes are capable of wonderful expression; and there is a hazel eye with a tinge of green in it, which is singularly handsome. Hazel eyes, matching with chestnut hair, are beautiful, and have the same velvety look which is so exquisite in black Oriental eyes.

"Black eyes," says Leigh Hunt, "are thought the brightest; blue the most feminine; grey the keenest. It depends entirely on the spirit within. We have seen all these colours change characters; though we must own that when a blue eye looks ungentle, it seems more out of character than the extremist contradiction expressed by the others."

Then there is a purple-blue eye, resembling the leaf of a pansy, which is very beautiful.

The Greeks admired large eyes—"Ox-eyed" is an epithet applied by Homer to Juno—and large eyes *are* very beautiful when they are not too prominent, and have enough expression. The almond-shaped long eye is very handsome, and so is that finely-shaped orbit we see on Greek statues. It is both handsome and intellectual.

But, after all, the eye derives its chief beauty

from expression, and, whether brilliant velvety black, or hazel, or violet, or heavenly blue, is still merely bead-like, if it does not express the informing soul of intelligence and love. The more intellectual and the kinder a woman is, the more lovely her eyes must inevitably grow.

> Eyes affectionate and glad,
> That seem to love whate'er they look on.
> CAMPBELL.

Small eyes require to be lit up by good nature and fun to be beautiful; but, thus lighted, are very charming.

Happily the eyes cannot be subjected to the destroying arts of the toilette, as the complexion and hair are. The only possible means of improving, or effecting a *fancied* improvement of, the eyes, is by darkening the edges of the lids by kohl; and this is so palpable that it can never deceive any one, and is therefore useless, when intended to deceive.

A bright natural colour on the cheek adds to the lustre of the eyes; but rouge gives them too strong a glare to be beautiful.

Good health will give lustre and clearness to them, and is, as in all other respects, essential to beauty.

The eyes should not be dimmed by reading by firelight or twilight, or by reading in bed. Early sleep adds to their brilliancy, and the nursery term of "beauty sleep," before midnight, is the popular acknowledgment of a great truth.

When the eyes have been tried by the glare of the sea, or the wind in them, when riding, it is well to bathe them with lukewarm rose-water, which is very good for the eyes at all times.*

The eyes should not be used on first waking for reading; nor indeed is it well to tax them before breakfast in any way. Bathe them well with cold water on rising. Never sit reading or working *facing* the light; let it fall on your work or book from behind you, or from the side. Nei-

---

* Ladies who read Greek, and at the same time care for their personal appearance (which we believe they will), should not try the eyes over it too long; and after reading, should bathe them with rose-water.

ther should the eyes be tried over minute stitches of needlework, or very small print.

These precautions will both preserve the beauty of the eyes and the precious gift of sight.

Any disease of the eyes should be instantly submitted to an experienced oculist.

We shall only add on the subject of eyes, that the expression being of so much importance, it is manifest that the more highly cultivated the intellect is, and the sweeter and happier the temper, the more chance the eyes have of being beautiful. A good expression will redeem even small and ill-shaped eyes from ugliness, and add a glory and depth to larger and more lustrous orbs.

The EYELASHES should be long, dark, and curling upwards. If cut in infancy they will grow long and thick; but cutting them afterwards is a fatal experiment, as they never grow long again. Large lids, which in a manner unroll over the eyes, are thought beautiful—perhaps because they imply large eyes; but such lids are very handsome. Care should be taken not to rub the eye so as to injure or rub out the lashes. The little gatherings on the edge of the lid, called sties, are very injurious to the lashes, and should be guarded against as much as possible. They imply, we believe, debility; and a doctor's advice and tonics might prevent them. When they exist, the best mode of treating them is to bathe them with warm water, or weak poppy-water. The old custom of rubbing them with a plain gold ring is not to be despised, as the pressure and friction excite the vessels of the lid, and cause an absorption of the suffused matter under the eyelash.

For all inflammations of the eye, we advise our readers at once to have recourse to medical advice.

The EYEBROWS should be finely marked, slightly arched, long and narrow; yet the narrow line should be thickly covered, so as to be well marked, as if pencilled. Too arched eyebrows give a silly look to the face.

> Upon her eyelids many graces sat
> Under the shadow of her even brows,

says Spenser. Shakspeare thought a certain

squareness of the brow beautiful. Describing a beautiful woman, he makes Pericles say,

> My queen's *square brows,*
> Her stature to an inch, as wand-like straight
> As silver voiced—her eyes as jewel-like,
> And *cased as richly ;*

i.e., set in beautiful, well-fringed orbits.

It is quite allowable to improve the growth of the eyebrows ; and it is quite possible to do so, by simply brushing them at night with a camel's-hair brush dipped in *cocoa-nut oil.* Every time the face is washed, the eyebrows should be very gently pressed into a curve by the thumb and finger.

Painting the eyebrows will make the skin rough and rubbly, and cause them, after a time, to fall off.

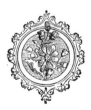

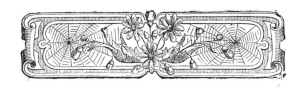

CHAPTER VI.

THE LOWER PART OF THE FACE.

The Ears—Ear-rings—Jaw—Cheeks—Nose—The mouth—Its
expression—Causes of its shape—Colour of the lips—Their
shape—The teeth—How to preserve them—The chin.

EAUTIFUL Ears are small, delicate,
and compact, of a shell-like shape,
and are thought indicative of high
birth. It has been observed that musicians have
frequently well-formed and small ears.

Ear-rings are the only mode of ornamentation
adopted for the ear, and most of our poets have
condemned their use; it seems, in truth, a re-
mainder of barbarism to make holes in the flesh
That the ear is actually disfigured by heavy

drops we think none of our ladies will deny. Sir
Philip Sidney says on this subject:

> The tip no jewel needs to wear:
> The tip is jewel of the ear.

And, however elegant they may be as ornaments,
we are inclined to be of his opinion about ear-
rings, thinking the tip the prettier when it has
never been pierced and pulled downwards by
heavy drops. When earrings are worn, they
should not be so heavy as to distort the ear itself.

The JAW should be small and delicate. A
large angular jaw gives a woman a masculine
appearance: it has a hard domineering look. In
a man it expresses resolution and perseverance,
and has a beauty of its own.

The CHEEK possesses great beauty, especially
in the transition from the lower part to the neck.
Dimpled cheeks have the charm of youth. Of
their colour we shall speak when we treat of the
complexion.

The NOSE has generally, in our nation, the
least claim to beauty. Mr. Disraeli has made

Sidonia call us "flat-nosed Franks," with some jus-
tice. The straight nose is the best shape—firmly
cut, and yet delicate; the Greek nose is especially
pretty in women; the Roman, or aquiline, a little
too hard-looking for female beauty, but still it
is handsome. A little turned-up nose is *piquant*,
arch, and pretty. Ordinary noses are not of themselves beautiful, and yet if we could replace one
which is of itself not pretty by a finely-cut one,
we should probably spoil the face, as the adaptation of the nose to the other features is the chief
thing. It is a feature for whose benefit we can
do nothing, but must perforce be compelled to
accept it as it is. We may add that it is a more
important feature in a man's face than a woman's.
Great dignity belongs to the male aquiline nose,
which has been possessed by most conquerors
and great warriors.

The most common nose amongst our young
English damsels is the *retroussé*. It cannot com-
pete with the Greek or aquiline nose, but it has
a special charm of its own. La Fontaine, describing a beautiful princess, says:

Une aimable et vive Princesse
A pied blanc et mignon, à brune et longue tresse,
Nez troussé, c'est un charme encore selon mon avis ;
C'en est même un des plus puissants.*

The MOUTH has been ranked next in beauty
to the eyes.   We are inclined to believe that its
charm is even greater ; for its expression is more
potent, for pleasing or displeasing, than that of
any other feature.   The rule—often beautifully
varied—is that the width of the mouth should
just equal the breadth of the nostrils, that the
lips should not make sharp angles, but keep a
certain breadth to the end, and show the red to
the last.   When, however, the nose is pinched
in, or very narrow, it is desirable that the mouth
should be much wider.   A large mouth is hand-
somer than one that is *too* small and pinched. A
pursed-up mouth is expressive of narrowness and
conceit.

The LIPS should be plump and full, according

---

* An amiable and brilliant Princess,
With small white foot and long brown tresses,
And *little turned-up nose*, her greatest charm.

to the hackneyed but still perfect picture drawn
by Sir John Suckling of the "Bride":

> Her lips were red, and one was thin,—
> Compared with that was next her chin,
> Some bee had stung it newly.

Very thin lips are ugly, because they express
meanness and bad temper. Chaucer says of the
lips,

> Lippës, thick to kiss percase;
> For lippës thin, not fat, but ever lean,
> They serve for naught, they be not worth a bean.
> "*Court of Love.*"

The lips and mouth are so much affected by
the habitual temper, that naturally thin lips will
grow full and less contracted by the simple in-
dulgence of frank and kindly feelings. Good
humour will always make a charming mouth.
Ill temper causes the corners of the lips to drop
downwards, and gives them the expression of
that feeling. Good temper and smiles curl the
lips upwards.

The mouth cannot practise disguise as the eyes
can. Whatever is our habitual character and temper, it writes itself indelibly on the lips. An ex-

quisitely-shaped mouth has no charm without
expression, and some mouths have little or none
beyond that of temper.   A smiling handsome
mouth is beautiful, or it will derive equal beauty
from an expression of pensive tenderness, pity,
or sympathy.

It is moral beauty which makes it beautiful.
Without it the mouth, peevish, scornful, sensual,
simpering, harsh, and cruel, is the worst, as it is
also the most truthful, feature in the face; while
the largest and plainest mouth may be made
pleasant, and even pretty, by kind sweet smiles
and a laugh which "rings from the soul."   The
red of the lips should be very rosy and brilliant;
it can scarcely be too vivid.

Paint is used, we believe, by some absurd women, on the lips—we need scarcely say to their
ultimate injury, and always at the user's peril.
The best way to colour the lips is to take care
of the health, on the goodness of which their
colour entirely depends.   The lips are infallible
as a test of health; though the very vivid painted-
looking red may sometimes be significant of
disease in the system.

Fresh rosy lips are the reward of not tightening the figure; of exercise, early rising, and temperate living. Good temper and cheerfulness give them their final charm of smiles and sweetness. Our harsh climate, however, tries the lips greatly in winter, and lip-salve is then allowable. It should be used at night. The following is a good receipt for it :—Two ounces of white wax, two ounces of olive oil, a quarter of an ounce of spermaceti, ten drops of oil of lavender, one ounce of alkanet root. Soak the alkanet for three days in the olive oil; then strain the oil, and melt the spermaceti and wax in it. When nearly cold, put in the oil of lavender, and stir it till quite firmly set.—From " Walsh's Domestic Economy."

But the finest-shaped mouths and the loveliest lips will be spoiled if the TEETH be bad.

Good teeth are the first essential of beauty. Can we imagine a beauty with black decayed teeth ? But how are good teeth to be obtained?— by dentifrices and brushing ? No! By simple washing, and a good digestion.

We cannot too earnestly urge on mothers the

necessity of attending *early* to the teeth of their children. We have known many cases in which the decay of the first teeth has caused the destruction of their more durable successors. First teeth, if they decay (as they sometimes do, from the infant's bad health or from difficulty of teething), should be soon removed, and not let remain till pushed out by the second teeth.

The cause of so much decay in the teeth now-a-days, is said by physicians to be the too great *whiteness* of our bread. Brown bread contains phosphates of wheat, essential for the preservation and nourishment—the building up, as it were—of the teeth ; and this has long been withheld from us in our daily bread. The teeth have suffered for it.

A very learned lawyer with whom we have the honour of being acquainted, and who uses his great intellect on ordinary as well as great matters, told us that he found all his children losing their teeth before they were fifteen, and he resolved to try what restoring the lost material of the teeth would do to save them. The children were not only made to eat brown bread (which contains the phosphates), but he gave them phosphates of wheat and lime-water, mixed in their tea or in water, and *at once* stopped the decay, as by a spell. Any chemist would direct the quantities to be taken by an adult. We recommend the trial of this remedy to all those whose teeth are giving signs of decay.

Perfect health—that great secret of beauty—is of course the cause of fine teeth.

The teeth should be of moderate size, even, and of a pearly white, with full enamel. Dead, dull white teeth have a very painful look.

Perfect cleanliness is essential to the preservation of the teeth. After every meal, whenever it is possible to leave the room, the mouth should be washed out, and the food removed from between the teeth by a quill toothpick. At night the teeth should be cleaned with a very soft brush of badger's hair; the ordinary hard brush scratches and cracks the enamel, and so causes decay. The water used should be lukewarm, but the mouth should be washed out with cold water afterwards, to strengthen the gums. No powder should be used but charcoal, which, if used about once or twice a week, will purify and clean the mouth. A little myrrh should occasionally be dropped into the water with which the gums are rinsed, to harden them. Soft spongy gums are apt to cause the teeth to decay at the root. Eau de Cologne should never be used for the teeth—it will make them brittle.

The inside of the teeth should be cleaned as carefully as the outside, and the gums should be rubbed also, but not up or down *from* the teeth.

On the slightest appearance of decay, or a tendency to accumulate tartar, or any derangement of the teeth, it is best to go at once to a dentist.

If a dark spot appears under the enamel, it is an indication of what is termed *caries :* neglect it, and the decay will eat in until it reaches the centre, and great agony is the sure result. But if a dentist sees the tooth at the first stage, removes the decayed part, and plugs the cavity in a proper manner, no farther mischief will result.

Tartar is not so easily dealt with, but it requires equally early attention. It results from an impaired state of the general health, and assumes the form of a yellowish concretion on the teeth and gums. At first, it is possible to keep it down by a repeated and vigorous use of the toothbrush, which for this purpose must be harder than a badgers' hair one ; but if a firm solid mass of tartar accumulates, it is necessary to have it chipped off by a dentist. Unfortunately, too, by that time it will probably have begun to loosen and destroy the teeth on which it fixes, and is pretty certain to have produced one obnoxious effect—that of tainting the breath.

About toothache, it is only necessary to point out that it results from various causes, and that, therefore, it is impossible to give any general remedy for it. It may be occasioned by decay, by inflammation of the membrane covering the fang, or the pain may be neuralgic, or there may be other causes.

Where there is inflammation, relief is often gained by applying camphorated chloroform, to be procured at the chemist's. This has often succeeded when laudanum and similar applications have entirely failed.

Neuralgia can only be attacked by means of quinine. It often assails those whose teeth are perfectly sound—affecting the nerves, and it is always to be distinguished, from the fact that the paroxysms of pain occur at regular intervals. Quinine is the only effectual remedy.

The following receipts for tooth-powder have been found useful, though charcoal alone is sufficient, and to be preferred to all others.

Rye Tooth-powder.—Rye contains carbonate of lime, carbonate of magnesia, oxide of iron, manganese, and silica—all suitable for application to the teeth. Therefore a fine tooth-powder is made by burning rye or rye bread to ashes, and grinding it to powder by passing the rolling-pin over it. Pass the powder through a sieve, and use. The crumbs of a French roll, though not so good, may be treated in the same way.

Camphorated Chalk.—This favourite tooth-powder is easily made. Take a pound of prepared chalk, and with this mix two drachms of campho-

very finely powdered, and moisten with spirits of wine. Thoroughly mix.

Remedy for Toothache.—Oil of cloves, four drops; chloroform, one drachm; eau de Cologne, one drachm; solution of acetate of morphia, two drachms; one grain to a drachm. Mix for a lotion for cold in the teeth and gums; to be applied with a camel's-hair pencil.—E. H.

We close our remarks upon the mouth with the following charming translation made from Ariosto by Leigh Hunt:

> Next, as between two little vales, appears
> The mouth, where spices and vermilion keep;
> There lurk the pearls, richer than sultan wears,
> Now casketed, now shown by a sweet lip;
> Thence issue the soft words and courteous prayers,
> Enough to make a churl for sweetness weep;
> And there the smile taketh its rosy rise,
> That opens upon earth a paradise.

The CHIN should be round and cushiony, turning a little upward, but not too much, or in age it is apt to become nut-crackerish by meeting the nose. A sharp projecting chin gives an old look to the face. A retreating chin has an air of silliness. A dimple in the chin is a great beauty.

Occasionally a sort of soft down like a moustache is seen on the upper lip of dark beauties. This is thought handsome, and gives great expression to the countenance.

We have now chatted about the figure and features of Beauty, it remains to discuss that all-important subject, the Complexion, which we shall reserve for another chapter.

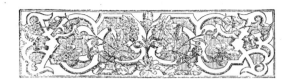

CHAPTER VII.

COMPLEXION.

British complexions—Cosmetics—Scripture notice of painting the face—Danger of white paint and rouge—Milk as a cosmetic—Nature of the skin explained—How to preserve it—Soft water—Effects of hard water and soap—Hot water—Cold water—Animal grease—Oil—Violet powder—Early rising—Receipts.

THE British have been for centuries famed for beauty of COMPLEXION. A bad complexion in healthful youth is the exception to the rule for British women. And yet we have recently read that the use of cosmetics was introduced into modern Europe by the English! Perhaps their appreciation of their valuable national gift led them to imitation in cases where it was lacking; but the use of cosmetics has been common in all ages and in every land. Scripture itself records the painting of Jezebel; and Ezekiel the prophet speaks of the eye-painting common among the women, and Jeremiah of *rending* the face with painting —a most expressive term for the destruction of beauty by such means. For the surest destroyers of real beauty are its simulators; the usurper destroys the rightful sovereign.

One thinks with a shudder of horror of Jeremiah's words, when one remembers how one of the beautiful Gunnings, whose native complexion was unrivalled, not only destroyed it by paint, but actually died at twenty-eight years of age, of cancer in the face, caused by her use of pigments.

That paint can ever deceive people, or really add to beauty for more than the duration of an acted charade or a play, when "distance lends enchantment to the view," is a delusion; but it is one into which women of all times and nations have fallen, from the painted Indian squaw to the rouged and powdered denizen of Paris or London.

Milk was the favourite cosmetic of the ladies of ancient Rome. They applied plasters of bread and ass's milk to their faces at night, and washed them off with milk in the morning. Poppœa, the wife of Nero, was wont to bathe in ass's milk.

As a cosmetic, milk would be harmless; but we doubt its power of improving the skin. As a beverage, no doubt it whitens the complexion more than any other food.

But before we speak of improving the complexion, it will be well to explain to our readers the nature and properties of the skin.

This is what an American physician has recently told us about it:

" Physiologically considered, it would seem almost impossible to over-estimate the importance of its functions. Consider for a moment the complex apparatus by which these functions are carried on, and the enormous amount of work accomplished through it. If the reader will examine his hand with a simple jeweller's lens, or with any of the cheap pocket microscopes, he will notice that there are delicate grooves crossing the furrows, and that a small orifice exists in the centre of each of them. Some of these orifices occupy nearly the whole of the groove, and are the openings of the perspiratory ducts, from which may be seen to issue, when the hand is warm, minute shining dots of perspiratory matter.

"But perspiration is not held in the body as water is held in a sponge, which can be squeezed out by pressure or by throwing it about; neither does it exist ready formed within us, as are the juices in apples and oranges. Upon the under surface of the true skin there are a multitude of little cavities, and in them are minute *glands*, which resemble ravelled tubes, formed of basement membrane and epithelial scales, with true secreting surfaces. It is the work of these little organs to receive the impure blood which is constantly brought to them through a network of arteries, and to *purify* it; and to thrust out of the system the waste or offensive matter which is separated from it. These impurities come along

in the blood, and are cast out through the perspiratory ducts while dissolved in that medium.
After the blood is thus cleansed, another set of
vessels are ready at hand to carry it back into
the interior of the body, to become again and
again loaded with impurities, which the little
glands are tireless in extracting and removing.
What organs in the human body subserve higher
or more vital purposes than these? Does the liver
or the stomach, or do the kidneys or the lungs,
stand in more intimate relation with life than these
little glands? We think not. Their size varies in
different parts of the body. In the palm of the
hand they are from 1-1,000th to 1-2,000th of an
inch in diameter, while under the arm they are
1-60th of an inch. The length of the tube, which
constitutes both gland and duct, is about a quarter
of an inch, and the diameter is about 1-1,700th of
an inch. It is a curious fact that the ducts, while
traversing the true skin, are perfectly straight;
but as soon as they enter the tough scarf-skin,
they become spiral, and resemble a corkscrew, so
that the perspiration is propelled around the tube

several times before it is ejected. Now, we are talking about *small things ;* but so long as we confine our descriptions to a single duct, we utterly fail to realize their minuteness. Let us look at them collectively. On every square inch of the palm of your hand, reader, there are at least 3,500 *of these perspiratory ducts.* Each one of them being one quarter of an inch long, we readily see that every square inch of skin surface on this part of the body has seventy-three feet of *tubing*, through which moisture and effete matter are constantly passing, night and day. The ducts, however, are shorter elsewhere ; and it will be fair to estimate sixty feet as the average length of the ducts for each square inch of the body. This estimate (reckoning 2,500 square inches of surface for a person of ordinary size) gives for these ducts an aggregate length of twenty-eight *miles.*

"The amount of liquid matter which passes through these microscopical tubes in twenty-four hours, in an adult person in sound health, is about sixteen fluid ounces, or one pint. One ounce of

the sixteen is *solid* matter, made up of organic
and inorganic substances, which, if allowed to remain in the system for a *brief space* of time,
would cause death. The rest is water. Besides
the water and solid matter, a large amount of
carbonic acid, a gaseous body, passes through the
tubes ; so we cannot fail to understand that they
are *active workers*, and also we cannot fail to see
the importance of keeping them in perfect *working* order, removing obstructions by frequent
application of water, or by some other means.
Suppose we obstruct the functions of the skin
perfectly, by *varnishing* a person completely with
a compound impervious to moisture. How long
will he live? Not over six hours. The experiment was once tried on a child at Florence.
Pope Leo X., on the occasion of his accession to
the Papal chair, wished to have a living figure to
represent the Golden Age, and so he had a poor
child gilded all over with varnish and gold-leaf.
The child died in a few hours. If the fur of a
rabbit or the skin of a pig be covered with a solution of India-rubber in naphtha, the animal ceases

to breathe in a couple of hours. These state-ments are presented in order that we may obtain some idea of the importance of the functions of the skin." — "*Fireside Science,*" by James R. Nichols, M.D.

From this our fair readers may judge of the dangerous consequences to the health of painting white and red—using *assistance,* as the ladies' maids say. Happily only a portion of the skin suffers from this pernicious folly ; but even in that degree great harm is done, and the skin itself soon shrivels and turns yellow, compelling a per-sistence in the same habits long after they are desired by their victim.

Skins differ. Some are cold and smooth ; some moist and warm ; some oily ; some hard and dry. They differ also in thickness, colour, and elasticity. The thin, soft, and delicate skins belong to the brunettes, the thick to the dead white complexions. The grain of the skin also differs—it is fine or coarse, as it may be.

Now, how is the skin to be kept fine and beautiful? By perfect cleanliness, air, sunshine, and good health.

Sunshine, in spite of tanning and freckles, is good for the skin. So is fresh air. Both united give bloom and colour to it; and if the air and sunshine are taken early, before the former has lost its morning fragrance, and while the latter has not yet gained its power to tan, the benefit is very certain, and a bloom of Hebe may be expected.

Now about cleanliness. The skin should be washed all over daily, in a bath if possible. But sometimes baths are not easily attainable. The following substitute for them will be found effectual:

Have a small square cut from a *thick* blanket, put it before your wash-hand stand. Obtain a *very* large square sponge and a piece of soft flannel. Stand in a little luke-warm water in the foot-pan, which is to be placed on the blanket; soap all over with the flannel, and use the *best* soap you can buy. Water without soap will not cleanse you: the oil of the skin resists it. Wash off the soap. This washing should be done in warm water. Then fill the large sponge with cold water, and sponge all over for freshness. Dry your skin with a coarse towel, and rub long and hard, till the skin glows.

This system of washing the skin will preserve you in health during the whole winter; and many people who cannot bear the shock of a cold bath *can* bear the cold sponging after washing.

The water used for the skin should be rain-water; but if London rain-water, it must be filtered to clear it from smuts.

Hard water is most objectionable. The process of washing with it has been thus described by a learned professor:

"First, the skin is wetted with the water, then soap is applied; the latter soon decomposes all the hardening salts contained in the small quantity of water with which the skin is wetted, and there is then formed a strong solution of soap, which penetrates into the pores of the skin. This is the process which goes on whilst a lather is produced in washing, but now the lather requires to be removed from the skin. How can this be done? Obviously only in one of two ways, viz., by wiping it off with a towel or by rinsing it away with water. In the former case the pores of the skin are left filled with soap solution, in the latter they become plugged up with the greasy curdy matter which results from the action of the hard water upon the soap solution occupying the pores of the skin. As the latter process of removing the lather is the one universally adopted, the operation of washing with soap and hard water is perfectly analogous to that used by the dyer or calico-printer when he wishes to fix a pigment in the pores of any tissue. He first introduces into the tubes of the fibre of calico, for instance, a liquid containing one of the ingredients necessary for the formation of the insoluble pigment; this is then followed by another liquid current containing the remaining necessary ingredients; the insoluble pigment is then produced within the very tubes of the cotton fibre, and is thus imprisoned in such a manner as to defy removal by subsequent washing. The pro-

cess of washing, therefore, in hard water, is es-
sentially one of dyeing the skin with the white,
insoluble, greasy and curdy salts of the fatty acids
contained in soap. The pores of the skin are thus
blocked up, and it is only because the insoluble
pigment produced is white, that such a repulsive
operation is tolerated. To those, however, who
have been accustomed to wash in soft water, the
abnormal condition of the skin thus induced is,
for a long time, extremely unpleasant."

When rain-water cannot be procured, the soap
should be washed off with *very warm* water,
which cleans the skin best.

Miss Nightingale has admirably explained the
effect of hot water on the skin.

"Compare," she says, "the dirtiness of the
water in which you have washed when it is cold
without soap ; cold with soap ; hot with soap.
You will find the first has hardly removed any
dirt at all ; the second a little more ; the third a
great deal more. But hold your hand over a cup
of hot water for a minute or two, and then, by
merely rubbing with your finger, you will bring

off flakes of dirt or dirty skin. After a vapour bath you may peel your whole self clean in this way. What I mean is, that by simply washing or sponging with water you do not really clean your skin. Take a rough towel, dip one corner in very hot water,—if a little spirit be added to it, it will be more effectual,—and then rub as if you were rubbing the towel into your skin with your fingers. The black flakes which will come off will convince you that you were not clean before, however much soap and water you have used. These flakes are what require removing. And you can really keep yourself cleaner with a tumbler of hot water and a rough towel and rubbing, than with a whole apparatus of bath and soap and sponge, without rubbing. It is quite nonsense to say that anybody need be dirty.

"Washing, however, with a large quantity of water, has quite other effects than those of mere cleanliness. The skin absorbs the water and becomes softer and more perspirable. To wash with soap and soft water is, therefore, desirable from other points of view than that of cleanliness."

A hot bath occasionally is very desirable, but when it cannot be had, washing in the manner we have described, may take its place.

The cold bath, when people can bear it, is health-giving and invigorating, but *not* cleansing. Sea-water baths are still less useful in the way of cleansing; indeed, a warm bath is often found necessary after a short course of them. The same remark applies to the sea-salt baths now so much in vogue. Apart from the invigorating effect of the cold water in the daily bath, the friction occasioned by the rub of the towel is very beneficial. Rough towels should therefore be used in moderation.

Milk baths, and baths impregnated with perfumes, need not be mentioned except as absurdities in which silly women have believed and still do believe; but they are too expensive for the general public to be guilty of such folly.

The use of eau de Cologne occasionally in the water used for washing the face and neck will be very desirable, as it assists in cleansing and brightening the skin; or a little gin may be used instead of eau de Cologne.

Elderflower-water cools and refreshes, and therefore benefits the skin; so also does rose-water, but scarcely with as good results. In summer the use of these perfumed and spirituous waters will be found very pleasant and freshening, and is quite allowable.

But animal grease of any kind, and *cold cream*, should never be put near the skin.

If greasing it is required, olive oil should be used, and this will sometimes be beneficial for very dry chapped skins, as it softens them. Rub the face with it gently every night in winter, and your skin will never chap.

But a naturally oily skin must on no account have oil used for it; a few drops of camphor in water may be used, or it may be powdered with fuller's earth, after washing, as a baby's skin is sometimes treated. Violet powder constantly used makes the skin rough, and enlarges the pores.

Neither paint (which, as we have seen, may produce terrible diseases, and can only harm the skin), nor powder, nor grease, are necessary.

Rain-water, good soap, and a rough towel suffice
for a perfect toilette.

We subjoin a quotation from some excellent
articles on this subject which appeared in "Land
and Water" some two or three years ago. They
were called the "Secrets of Beauty." The pas-
sage to which we allude is *à propos* of one of the
famous beauties of the sixteenth century.

"It was not to such tricks"—the writer has
been speaking of wearing masks, and of Margue-
rite de Navarre's quarrel with her husband, Henri
Quatre, who objected to her sleeping in one
—"It was not to such tricks that Diana of
Poitiers, Duchess of Valentinois, resorted to preserve her beauty to the age of threescore years
and ten ; she who at sixty-five rode on horseback
like a girl ! This remarkable woman was a cele-
brated beauty in an age of beauties, yet, strange
to say, no historian has ever given details of those
wondrous charms which captivated two kings,
one of them fifteen years her junior in age. We
do not even know whether her eyes were blue or
black, whether her hair was light or dark ; we

only know that she was the loveliest woman at
a Court of lovely women, and that at an age
when most women are shrivelled specimens of
ugliness. People said she possessed a secret that
rendered her thus impervious to the ravages of
time. Some went so far as to say in that super-
stitious age that she had bought her secret from
a very dark gentleman indeed! What was this
secret, then? Did she ever tell it? Never. Did
any one ever know it? Yes, her perfumer. Did
he never tell it? Not during her life. It is
known, then? It is, for those who have the
patience to wade through musty manuscripts and
books. May we not know it? You will only
smile and disbelieve! Try. Good, then, I will
translate Maître Oudard's own words to you:—
'I, Oudard, apothecary, surgeon, and perfumer,
do here declare on my faith and on the memory
of my late honoured and much-beloved mistress,
Madame Diane of Poitiers, Duchess of Valentinois, that the only secret she possessed, with
which to be and remain in perfect health, youth,
and beauty to the age of seventy-two, was—*rain*

water ! And, in truth, I assert there is nothing in the world like this same rain-water, a constant use of which is imperative to render the skin soft and downy, or to freshen the colour, or to cleanse the pores of the skin, or to make beauty last as o ng as life ! '

"Thus, the only service which Maître Oudard rendered his illustrious mistress was to gather the rain-water for her, bottle it and seal it up, to be in readiness in case of scarcity of rain. So all these bottles of *philtres* which daily arrived from the great perfumer to the still greater lady only contained *rain-water !* Is that possible ?

"Diana always took an hour's outdoor exercise before the dew had left the ground."

Early rising is no doubt one of the secrets of beauty ; that it was so understood by our ancestors, the superstition of the May dew testifies. But now, alas ! the attendant spirits of our households will never rise till the dew has long evaporated. For our young ladies early rising soon becomes a forgotten virtue of the school-room.

Moles are frequently a great disfigurement

to a face, but they should not be tampered with in any way. The only safe and certain mode of getting rid of them is by a surgical operation.

Freckles are of two kinds. Those occasioned by exposure to the sunshine, and consequently evanescent, are denominated "summer freckles;" those which are constitutional and permanent are called "cold freckles."

With regard to the latter, it is impossible to give any advice which will be of value. They result from causes not to be affected by mere external applications.

Summer freckles are not so difficult to deal with, and with a little care the skin may be kept free from this cause of disfigurement.

Some skins are so delicate that they become frecked on the slightest exposure to the open air in summer. The cause assigned for this is, that the iron in the blood, forming a junction with the oxygen, leaves a rusty mark where the junction takes place.

If this be so, the obvious cure is to dissolve the

combination—for which purpose several courses have been recommended.

1. At night wash the skin with elderflower-water, and apply this ointment—made by simmering gently together one ounce of Venice soap, a quarter of an ounce of deliquated oil of tartar, and ditto of oil of bitter almonds. When it acquires consistency, three drops of rhodium may be added. Wash the ointment off in the morning with rose-water.

2 (and best). One ounce of alum, ditto of lemon-juice, in a pint of rose-water.

3. Scrape horseradish into a cup of cold sour milk, let it stand twelve hours, strain, and apply two or three times a day; but this remedy is painful, and must be used with care.

4. Mix lemon-juice, one ounce; powdered borax, a quarter of a drachm; keep for a few days in a glass bottle; apply occasionally.

5. Another remedy is, muriate of ammonia, half a drachm; lavender-water, two drachms; distilled water, half a pint; apply two or three times a day.

6. Into half a pint of milk squeeze the juice of a lemon, with a spoonful of brandy, and boil, skimming well; add a drachm of rock-alum.

There are various other discolorations of the skin, proceeding frequently from derangement of the system ; the cause should always be discovered before attempting a remedy, otherwise you may increase the complaint instead of curing it.

Mr. Wilson recommends the following as a good cerate for removing discoloration of the skin :

"Elderflower ointment, one ounce ; sulphate of zinc, twenty grains ; mix well, and rub into the affected skin at night. In the morning wash it off with plenty of soap, and when the grease is completely removed, apply the following lotion : infusion of rose-petals, half a pint ; citric acid, thirty grains. All local discolorations will disappear under this treatment ; and, if the freckles do not entirely yield, they will, in most instances, be greatly ameliorated. Should any unpleasant irritation, or roughness of the skin, follow the application, a lotion composed of half a pint of almond mixture and half a drachm of Goulard's extract, will afford immediate relief."

In conclusion, we may sum up the whole matter of personal beauty by saying it is produced chiefly by good health, early rising, leaving the figure uncompressed, and being intelligent and good-tempered.

A placid temper will long keep wrinkles in abeyance, and years of good humour and kindness will leave a sweet mouth to old age, while cultivated intelligence will give expression and spirit to the eyes.

Thus we see that goodness and sense are the best handmaids of beauty, and that "beautiful for ever" may not be a dream and a delusion. Of a beautiful woman thus embellished and preserved, we may say with Shakspeare's Miranda,

Sure nothing ill can dwell in such a temple.

We must say a few words about the disfigurement to which the skin is subject at times, in small black specks—a sort of pimple. A doctor informs us that these are caused by the enlargement of the perspiratory ducts, which leave a portion of the perspiring matter exposed to the air, which turns it black. It should be squeezed out; and if the tube is still large, and the same appearance likely to return, it must be touched *by a doctor* with caustic, to contract the opening; but, ordinarily, the duct will close of itself.

Small pimples may be removed by using a wash of about as much borax as would cover sixpence, in a cup of water: the face to be dabbed with it with a soft rag.

Gruel may be used to wash the face in cases of eruption, instead of soap, which will irritate the skin when not in a healthy condition; but in such cases resort should be had *at once* to the surgeons who have made the study of the skin a speciality, and no quack remedies should be used. All a lady can do for herself under the circumstances would be to use great cleanliness, and be careful not to wear any part of the dress tight.

Cosmetics destroy and never really improve the skin, whether it be in a healthy state or not.

Sallowness belongs to a bad state of health,

and should also come under the discipline of the physician.

The following simple receipts for the toilette appearing to be of use, we have given them a place in this chapter.

Toilet Vinegar.—Add to the best malt vinegar half a pint of cognac and a pint of rose-water. Scent may be added ; and if so, it should be first mixed with the spirit before the other ingredients are put in.

Philocome. — This is the name of a good French pomade. It is made by melting three ounces of white wax, by the action of hot water round the vessel in which it is placed, and while the heat is kept up adding a pound of olive oil. Scents, such as bergamot, may be added as the other ingredients cool. Varieties of perfumes are used by the manufacturers.

Sticking Plaster.—Stretch a piece of black silk on a wooden frame, and apply dissolved isinglass to one side of it with a brush. Let it dry ; repeat process, and then cover it with a strong tincture of balsam of Peru.

Lavender-Water.—This mildest of perfumes is a preparation of oil of lavender, two ounces, and orris root, half an ounce; put it into a pint of spirits of wine and keep for two or three weeks before it is used. It may require straining through blotting paper of two or three thicknesses.

Milk of Roses.—This is a cosmetic. Pound an ounce of almonds in a mortar very finely, then put in shavings of honey soap in a small quantity. Add enough rose-water to enable you to work the composition with the pestle into a fine cream; and in order that it may keep, add to the whole an ounce of spirits of wine by slow degrees. You may scent with otto of roses. Strain through muslin. Apply to the face with a sponge or a piece of lint.

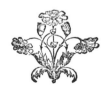

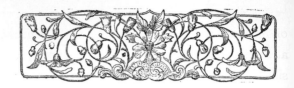

CHAPTER VIII.

DRESS WITH RESPECT TO BEAUTY.

Power of dress on beauty—Fashion—Why so imperative—Long-
past fashions—Form and colour—M. de Chevreul on colour
—Its effect on the complexion—Lace, a grey colour—Size
affected by colour—Stripes—Throat : shortened or length-
ened—Adaptations of dress to different ages.

E believe that few of our readers will
deny the truth of our assertion when
we say that beauty is not always, when
"unadorned, adorned the most;" in fact, in spite
of the poets, we believe that dress has much to
do with personal loveliness. It can enhance and
set off beauties and conceal defects in a much
greater degree than the generality of people are
aware of. FORM and COLOUR in conjunction, and
modified by fashion, are the materials of the art

of picturesque dress as well as of beauty. We advisedly say *picturesque*—by it we mean nothing singular or *outré*, but that skilful adaptation of *form* and *colour* which would best serve the artist if he were to be called on to paint a portrait of the wearer.

Fashion *must* be studied. Anything *just become old-fashioned* will always disagreeably affect the eye—probably, as we have said before, from association. We do not see the best people so dressed ; style is lacking, and the effect becomes mean and poor. The fashions of past centuries have not this effect on us. We connect them in imagination with the pictures in which we have seen them worn by the great and beautiful of past ages, and we admire them, and even wear them as becoming and ornamental when a fancy ball gives us the opportunity to do so. But with modern "old fashions" it is very different. No one can deny the singular fact that nearly everything fashionable is pleasing. The extreme of all fashions should, however, be avoided.

Happily, those of the present day lend themselves to picturesque effect; and in one point we may always use, in a great measure, our own taste and judgment—I mean in the matter of *colour*.

Now, of the secrets of *colour*, our women are too generally ignorant, though a move in the right direction has been made by the recent art-teaching, which is having its effect. Monsieur de Chevreul,-the superintendent of the Gobelin Tapestry manufacture, has, of late years, given us much information on this subject. He tells us that—

"Colours placed in juxtaposition effect a modification in tint or hue on each other. Place blue and green of nearly the same height of tone side by side, and you will perceive that the blue will look less greenish and become more violet, and the green will take an orange tinge."

"Under similar conditions, an orange and a red mutually affect each other, and pass respectively towards yellow and crimson. Even two white stripes by the side of two black, or even two grey stripes matched with two brown ones, undergo severally, and severally induce, a change, the tone of the grey or the brilliancy of the white being heightened, those of the brown and of the black being in a corresponding degree lowered by the mutual neighbourhood of these different stripes. It is then a phenomenon affecting tone (*i.e.,* relative depth of greyness) as well as tint (*i.e.,* relative quantity of colour). Furthermore, black, white, or grey, placed in juxtaposition with coloured stripes, exhibit changes, the character of which can be readily anticipated by reference to Chevreul's law. Thus, white with red mutually produce difference both in tone and tint. The *tone* of white (absolute whiteness being the greatest height of tone to which all colour can approximate) reacts on the tone of the red, lowering it. The *colour* of the red reacts on the colourlessness of the white, impressing this with a slight tint, not of red, dear reader, but of the colour most different from the red—that is to say, the complimentary colour, namely, *green.* Thus red and white become respectively a deeper-toned (darker) red contrasted with a slightly greenish

white. Thus, too, black and red become a very
faintly greenish and much less rich black, and a
more white (lower-toned, paler) red. The hue
variations become marvellously distinct in a well-
chosen grey whose tone is commensurate with
that of the colour juxtaposed to it. Here, the
modification of tone not affecting the relative
brilliancy of the colour and the grey, the former
impresses on the latter its complementary tint,
so that a red will render a like-toned grey quite
perceptibly green, itself becoming of a purer
redness, while a blue similarly brightened will
impart to it a decided orange. Greys slightly
tinted with any colour have that colour in a sur-
prising way intensified by juxtaposition with its
complementary, so that a bluish grey will become
almost a decided blue in the neighbourhood of
orange." *

The effect of colour in juxtaposition to the
complexion has, therefore, to be considered. We
have seen above that red placed against white

---

* "Fraser's Magazine," 1846.

gives the white a tinge of green. Our readers will understand, therefore, that although the skin is never a pure *white*, as silk or linen may be, still, red placed against it would not be becoming to a very fair complexion. A fair infant can scarcely bear the juxtaposition of a decided scarlet.

The rule is, you see, that the colour in juxtaposition will cast its *complementary* colour on the skin. But what are the complementary colours? We will explain.

There are three primary colours: red, blue, and yellow. These united form all the other colours—for example:

Red and blue form purple.

Red and yellow, orange.

Blue and yellow, green.

Now, each primary colour has its complementary colour in the *other two mixed together*. For instance: red has green for its complementary, because blue and yellow, the two other primary colours, make green. The complementary of yellow is *purple*, because red and blue make purple. Thus the effect of yellow, if placed in juxtaposition to a very *white* skin, would be to give it a tint of purple.

The complementary of blue is orange, for red and yellow make that colour. Thus we see that red would give a tint of green, yellow of purple, and blue of orange.

The secondary colours formed by the primary are *green*, made by the union of blue and yellow; *purple*, formed from red and blue; and *orange*, the union of red and yellow. The complementaries of these colours are the primaries themselves.

The secondary colours united form the greys, which are tinged with the hue of the colours which formed them. Thus we have a red grey, a blue grey, a greenish grey, a purple grey, &c. And then follow all the neutral tints, with the browns of many shades, the doves, stones, and fawn colours.

It will be apparent to our readers, at once, that the strong primary colours, placed in juxtaposition to the skin, cannot be very becoming, unless softened or modified. This is best done by the intervention of grey, which colour is given by *lace*, the white threads of which reflect light, while the spaces absorb it, and thus produce a grey shade.

White lace or black lace interposed between a strong colour and the skin will be found to produce a softening and harmonizing effect. It is possible that an instinctive sense of this fact has inclined milliners to make their bonnets more becoming by edging the strings which touch the chin and cheeks with lace.

The reflection of colour is another thing. A red light falling on the face would give a rosy tint—as we see in the effect of pink hangings to rooms, or the reflection of coloured glass. But in the present day there is little possibility of obtaining by dress a reflected colour on the face. When the bonnets surrounded the face, a pink lining would give a pretty rosy flush to it; but, now-a-days, bonnets cast no reflection, and the strings alone test the skill of the wearer, being in juxtaposition with the sides of the face. Hats, however, may still be studied with a view to the effect of reflection.

In speaking of colour, we must remember the infinite variety of tints, hues, and shades, all bearing the same generic name merely modified by an uncertain adjective. In nothing is language so wanting as in a nomenclature for colours. Blue—but how many shades of blue there are! Warm blues, colder blues, grey blues, lilac blues —no end of blues! We call them all by one name, yet the *tint* may make all the difference.

"The learned," says Alphonse Karr, whose wonderful bouquets prove how fully he understood the subject—"the learned who have invented so many words, ought to have imagined some that might give an exact idea of colours and their shades. * * * There are but few words to designate colours, and even they are taken at hazard from ideas that are very far removed from each other. This annoys me the more because colours have for me harmonies as ravishing as those of music—because they awaken in my mind thoughts perfectly strict and indivi-

dual, and their influence acts powerfully on my
imagination. It often happens, even in houses in
which I am not very much at home, that I rise
in the midst of a conversation to go and separate
two inimical colours which some unlucky chance
has brought into conjunction on one piece of
furniture. There are for me between colours and
their shades discords as strong as can possibly
exist between certain notes of music.

"There are no false colours except in the nomenclature of our *marchandes des modes;* but
there are assemblages of colours as false as the
notes of any one who had never had a bow in
his hand, but took up a violin and scraped away
at random. I remember two persons who were
always disagreeable to me on account of the
colours they persisted in wearing. The first was
a certain large woman, who always appeared in
green dresses and yellow bonnets; the other, a
man who decked himself out in staring red waist-
coats and bright blue cravats. I endeavoured to
contend against the prejudices inspired by such
disfigurements. I have reason to repent; I have

since had much to complain of in my relation with those two persons."

Monsieur Karr ends by proposing that colours should be defined by the names of flowers, as —Forget-me-not Blue, Westeria Blue, Bugloss Blue, &c.,—a plan of which we highly approve.

Using, however, our present nomenclature, we would say that turquoise blue is very becoming (in juxtaposition) to rather faded or very pale complexions; while the bugloss blue (darker and warmer) suits the fresh complexions or the warm brunette.   Blue is a comparatively cold colour, and suits nearly everybody.

Scarlet requires a warm brunette skin, which will look clearer for a tinge of green. Rose-colour is also very becoming to brunettes.

A paler pink will harmonize with a very fresh young complexion.

For the sallow, and those who are no longer young, pink is sadly trying—it mocks their want of bloom.

Amber suits warm brunettes and dark-haired people, but should be avoided by yellow-haired fair ladies, for whom a light pretty green or a tender blue is infinitely becoming.

Light green gives, in juxtaposition to white, a pink tinge.

But we must remember, as we have said, that the skin is never *quite* white—it is more or less flesh-colour; and this has to be considered when we think of the juxtaposition of colours. The best plan is personal experience. Every individual's complexion differs from others in some hue or tint, which must be nameless. Let every one try separately the effect of different colours against her skin, and suit it herself. Our present aim in these general hints is to show how important colours are in their effects, and how necessary it is to study them.

We will, then, merely add that violet, which is a modification of purple, gives a yellow tint to the skin, and is becoming to no complexion. Dead white is becoming to too-florid people, as it deadens the red colour by juxtaposition, but it makes p ale fade people look paler still.

Black, being the absence of colour, makes the

skin look whiter, as it impresses no tint on it, and is generally becoming, though undoubtedly young fresh-looking people sometimes do not look well in black.

The neutral tints also are very trying to faded complexions; they too nearly approach the colour of the skin, and give a washed-out look, deadening the complexion still more. Some of the brown tints, especially the chestnut browns, suit fair warm complexions *very* well. The colour of the hair is sure to become the skin.

The proportion of colour has also to be considered. A greater quantity of blue may be worn than of red or yellow. The proportion in light which produces perfect harmony of colour is nearly double blue to red, and eight parts of blue to three of yellow.

Brilliant colours relieving masses of dove, stone, grey, or black and brown, are very effective, and light up the wearer, as it were, with gleams of coloured light, without effacing her by their splendour, as they would do if worn in quantities.

Jewels should also be worn with regard to colour. Rubies do not look well with mauve, nor topazes with red; while pearls and mauve are exquisite together, and rubies show best with pearl-colour and *some* tints of green. Diamonds, from their lustre of many hues, may be worn with nearly every colour, but show best with black.

A general knowledge of the effect of colour will, we are sure, do much for harmony in dress.

Of colours worn in the hair, we may add that they should be brilliant and effective, harmonizing or in contrast. In red or auburn hair a pink bow should not be worn; green is the contrasting colour, and blue looks well in it.

In black hair, red, amber, light green, or a strong blue, looks well. In fair hair, light cerulean blue, deep rose-colour, or a strong green, will do.

White flowers do not look well in very light hair; colours are better. In pale brown hair crimson ribbon does well, or dark blue. Brunettes may wear the more brilliant colours, and will look the fairer for them. But we advise them to put lace *always* next the skin.

Considering colours with regard to dress, we would advise that the great body of colour should not be a strong and brilliant one, as scarlet, violet, bright green, &c.—unless it is very much softened down by dark trimmings. The dress should frame a picture, not withdraw attention from it to itself. But soft diaphanous dress may be of bright colours, supposing that the *hue* be very delicate.

With regard to the putting of colours together, Chevreul says, and truly, "When two tones of the same colour are juxtaposed"—laid side by side or next to each other—"the light colour will appear lighter and the dark colour darker." This applies in respect to light and dark; but the same will obtain in reference to *different* colours; thus a blue placed next to an orange will have the effect of giving power to both, for the orange will be more positively orange and the blue more positively blue, by what he—Chevreul—calls simultaneous contrast. The same holds with neutrals or tertiaries, contrasted with primaries or secondaries. A red ribbon on any very dark ground—say black—would appear light, while the same tint of red on a very light or white ground would appear much darker. Any colour in juxtaposition with its complementary must be heightened by such position, as must the complementary, reciprocally, in the same degree by the primary which is *its* complementary. This knowledge may be of great use in arranging a lady's toilette.

There are some peculiarities about colours besides this; blue and white have a singular power of apparently increasing size, consequently they should not be worn by stout figures.

Black apparently diminishes size, as do the browns and darker tones of green and crimson.

There is something very restless in yellow. The eye cannot remain pleasantly fixed on any mass of it; beyond a trimming, a ribbon, or a flower, it should be used with great judgment. But softened and toned down by being partially covered with black lace, it is effective, handsome, and well suited to brunettes.

Brown bears trimming with it in a dark or

amber shade, and is the only colour we like to see united to it.

Black and amber look well together.

We must say a word here as to the effect of colours with regard to the idea of warmth. It is a physical fact that some are really warmer—*i.e.,* absorb more heat—than others. Black, violet, indigo, and crimson are warm colours; green, blue, yellow, white are cold—therefore adapted for summer wear. The greys are warm or cold, according to the tint : a reddish grey would be warm, a blue grey cold.

Colours also should be worn in due proportion of harmony, and, as we have said before, the *mass* of colour in a dress should not be of brilliant hue. The blacks, browns, greys, stones, dove-colours are all better for the whole of the dress than the reds, blues, greens, or ambers, unless the latter are subdued by darker trimmings or some part of the dress being black ; but we think, for the due display of beauty, the less prominent hues, with gleams of brilliant colour united to them are best.

Lines affect the apparent height or breadth of the wearer. Stripes or trimmings down a dress give the appearance of greater height. Stripes or rows of trimming *round* the figure make it appear plumper *and shorter*. Consequently, too tall and too thin people should not wear stripes or trimmings down the dress but *round* it, and the dress should be full and bunchy.

Short and stout people should wear long dresses not much trimmed above the bottom of the skirt. Lines or trimmings should run downwards for them.

The waist of short ladies should not be worn too long, whatever the fashion may be, as it gives them a wasp-like look. Too great length of throat —especially when it is thin and scraggy—may be made less perceptible by wearing the hair full and low at the back of the neck. The dress should be made high at the throat, and a ruff or velvet should be worn ; or for evening dress a necklace. A throat too short and thick, which brings the head too near the shoulders, should have the hair raised at the back, and wear neither velvet nor necklace, but flat collars, and the dress cut low at the throat. We may observe here, *en passant*, that the thick white linen collars worn round the neck are unbecoming except to young ladies. The strong contrast of pure white is too trying for a complexion not in its first bloom; the soft grey of lace is much better in effect.

Much dignity is given by long and sweeping skirts, which also add to the apparent height of the figure. Short dresses make their wearers appear shorter; but, when fashionable, have a smart *piquant* look.

Light materials which have a certain airy grace about them, should be worn by young girls. It adds to their apparent age to dress in costly moirés, velvets, or dark rich silks, just as light airy dresses actually add in appearance to the age of their wearers when they are past youth. The transparent muslin or grenadine of brilliant green, mauve, or blue, which looks fairy-like and elegant on a young girl, gives an affected and *poor* look to her mother or aunt of maturer age.

More solid and richer materials, and richer, fuller

colours, belong to middle age, which has a ripe beauty of its own, and looks best in the brilliant hues of autumn, softened against the skin by lace, with which youth only can entirely dispense.

It is amazing how the study of an harmonious dress will bring out the Juno-like beauty of matrons, which is lost in the lightness of a more youthful attire. And for old age also, soft, dark, warm colours will do much—with plenty of lace to soften the faded skin and cover the silvery hair. For age, too, has its beauty, and it is incumbent on old ladies, as well as young ones, to make the most of all personal gifts. A more scrupulous cleanliness and a greater care as to what is worn, is needed in old age.

For rich old people black velvet, trimmed with old lace or fur, is always a becoming and beautiful dress; but there should always be gleams of rich colour about it—crimson, or bright rich blue, or violet in the costume somewhere. Old withered hands should have lace ruffles hanging *over* them, and should wear mittens.

The choice of colours and some thought in

blending them artistically will not take up more time than that bestowed on purchasing garments in bad taste—displeasing to the cultivated eye, and disfiguring to the wearer.

It is, therefore, surely not beneath the dignity of an English lady to take these matters into consideration.

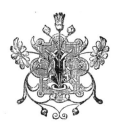

CHAPTER IX.

DRESS WITH RESPECT TO BEAUTY.

Gloves : fit, cut, length, colour—Boots : effect on size of foot—
   Artistic dress—The girl—The matron—the old lady.

THERE is no more complete finish to dress than a good glove. It should always be a shade lighter than the dress with which it is worn. Dark gloves with light dresses are in very bad taste.

Gloves should fit the hands perfectly; but there is little chance of this being effected except by having them made to measure. Every one who has been in Paris must remember the care with which the glover there tries on and fits her gloves. In England, where no trial of them is allowed, and the numbers are utterly uncertain, it is better to have gloves made for the hand, and this is done at some houses in London. An Irish lady of rank also employs girls in Ireland for this purpose, and thus enables them to earn an honest livelihood. Their gloves fit admirably.

The glove should be fully long enough to come over the wrist, and should have two or three buttons; otherwise the hand will look short and thick. An ill-fitting glove will, in fact, disfigure the most lovely hand. Gloves of the very palest shade of primrose, which look white by gaslight, are more becoming than the dead white kid, and last longer.

Gloves in former ages were embroidered with pearls and gems, and were costly property. Now-a-days, the excellence of their fit and their perfect freshness are their beauty.

French gloves are considered the best cut, but the Irish gloves of which we have spoken are quite as good.

The Swedish kid glove, in its natural tan-colour, looks very well, but it very soon becomes soiled, and is certainly not economical. The best gloves are always in the end the cheapest.

Gloves sewn with colours make the hands look larger. Attention should also be paid to the boots worn, as their good or bad shape disfigure or display the beauty of the foot. They should be made *longer* than is absolutely necessary, as length of boot makes the foot appear slender. Walking books should be thick enough to keep the feet dry. Their thickness will add to the height of the figure, and give a good firm tread—not flat-footed, as thin house-shoes are apt to look.

We believe we have now pointed out fully what is the effect and value of dress on personal beauty. We shall conclude this branch of our subject with the following extract from "Scribner's Monthly" (a clever American periodical), as embodying our idea of what woman's dress ought to be :

"In examining a well-executed ideal painting containing a female figure, we perceive that there are no incongruities ; the subject has been carefully studied in mass and detail. Age, too, has been considered. A young girl is represented in bright tint of delicate materials, with airy graceful outlines, which veil without hiding the rounded contours of youth; the matron is more richly and gorgeously arrayed, while the redundancy of her figure is obscured by the dark colours and long heavy skirts of her robe; and the aged lady is well wrapped in warm and abundant folds of garments and mantles, which hide her shrivelled form. In well-drawn pictures we find that a woman's hair is arranged to define the natural contour of her head. In youth the hair falls backward and downward in waving and curling masses ; in mature womanhood it is coiled round the head ; in old age a silken hood or lace kerchief still follows the natural outline, and makes drapery about the shrivelled neck."

In concluding this chapter, we beg to remind our readers that *taste* in dress, as in every other art, is worth cultivation ; and that when its perfection has been attained by Englishwomen, much of the expense lavished on costly but unbecoming and tasteless dress will be spared, for they will become capable of inaugurating fashions themselves, and will learn how, at how little expense, good taste will improve their national beauty.

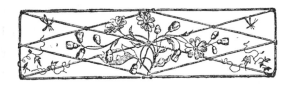

CHAPTER X.

CARE OF BEAUTY IN INFANCY.

Beauty to be thought of in infancy—Inseparable from health—
Preserving the complexion—Air, exercise, diet—Bath—
Light—Tanning and freckling; eyelashes—Teeth—Gums—
Figure—Walking—Reclining—Feet exercises—Hair—Eyes.

E cannot close our little treatise without a few words to mothers on the
importance of early taking into consideration the personal appearance of their children. And happily the subject leads to the
benefit not only of the beauty, but the health of
their babes, for without health there is no hope
of ultimate beauty.

All babes are lovely. If their features do
not promise perfection, their complexion, when
healthy, is beauty in itself. How clear and pure

the skin is! how bright and limpid the glance! how sweet and soothing the divine expression of purity and innocence!

That lovely complexion may be preserved, but, alas, seldom is! Our babes are too often shut up from the oxygen which should nourish the blood which forms their complexion, in close small nurseries; sometimes, in London, underground; and they sleep, in towns, too often in small ill-ventilated rooms, with the nurses.

Now, the first essential for a child's future beauty is ozone—that is, pure air and *plenty of it*, and sunshine. No nursery should look towards the north—it should have the morning sun, and it should be airy; and no child should sleep in a small bed-room with its nurse, with a smaller allowance of air than the law makes necessary in a national school. Give your babes oh mother! plenty of air and light, and they will grow like the flowers and be as lovely as they are.

But do not allow your little girls to freckle, for freckles are difficult to remove, and come early. They are caused by the oxygen in the air combining under the influence of sunshine ; they may be prevented by shading the face with the ordinary cotton sun-bonnet.

If the little face gets tanned, it will be worth washing it with elderflower-water at once. In fact, in summer it is sometimes needed to cool the skin.

Soft rain-water should always be used for infants, and never allow your nurse to be guilty of the dirty and skin-injuring process of bathing or washing two or three children in the same water. We are quite aware that this is never done in the higher-class nurseries ; but we believe it is too often the case in middle class ones. The water used should be *quite* pure and clean ; the soap of the very best kind—glycerine or honey soap, or the *very* best yellow, not that ordinarily used in washing ; but yellow soap is not pleasant on an infant's skin.

Exercise daily and good food are required for future beauty.

The mother may cut (carefully) the eyelashes of the sleeping infant (using scissors with two blunted points), and she will thus ensure long curled lashes by-and-bye. Every morning the wee nose should be caressingly streaked between the finger and thumb, to make it a good shape; and as the little girl grows older, her eyebrows may have a little cocoa-nut oil applied, if they appear to grow too thin and pale.

As the teeth grow they should be watched. They may be washed night and morning. Should the first teeth give signs of decay, the child should at once be taken to a *good* dentist for advice. Brown bread should always be given to children; they require it for the formation of bones and teeth, as it contains phosphates of wheat.

The gums (if the teeth threaten decay) should be bathed with weak myrrh and water. Examine also the diet, and ascertain that no sugar plums are given in the nursery. Pure white sugar will not hurt; but *bon-bons* are too often poisonous.

Watch the appearing of the second teeth. If they grow evenly, do not touch them; but if they are irregular, put them straight every day by gentle pressure. The pressure of a mother's tender finger will prevent much future expense and pain in dentistry. Never let your children—when the second teeth come—use hard toothbrushes; a small sponge and lukewarm water used after every meal is sufficient at first. When all are changed, a badger's hair toothbrush may be given to the child, and must be used occasionally or about once a day.

Stroke the eyebrows every morning into an arch.

With regard to the figure, we counsel you *never* to put the child in stays. Leave her as free in form as her brother, and she will be well-shaped and graceful. A looseish band of jean is sufficient to make her dress set smoothly. Do not permit a tight string anywhere; examine her dress daily yourself, for nurses are too careless in such matters.

Do not suffer her to sit without support to her back; encourage her to rest the spine by lying back in a chair; and once a day, after walking, make your children, both boys and girls, lie flat on the floor on a sheet for an hour. This will save weak spines, and make fine figures.

Children should not be made to sit still long at a time. If they are kept long in one place, they will fidget, move restlessly from side to side, and take attitudes which may make them grow crooked. Let then often march, and clap their hands, and raise arms as in infant schools—the training of which might be, with advantage, introduced into our nurseries.

The arm-exercises already suggested in this little book should be used after ten years of age; and no stooping lesson—such as writing a copy or bending over maps—should end without them. Accustom the children to walk about the room every day for about half an hour, with their arms crossed behind their backs and a book on their heads; and give a reward to the child who can soonest carry a basket or vase on her head without letting it fall.

Exercises with the feet are also good for children, and may be taught with advantage. They should never be suffered to do anything awk-

wardly without being shown how to do it better ;
but they must not be harassed with frequent
fault-finding or laughed at, or they will grow
shy, nervous, and *infallibly awkward*. Notice if
a child bites its nails, and check the habit at
once, as it utterly spoils both nails and fingers.

It is by careful watching in infancy and childhood that high-bred girls are made so lovely and
graceful; for beauty must be cared about, and
grace inculcated in the nursery, if we hope to see
its perfection in after years. When schoolroom
duties come, the same watchfulness cannot be so
well exercised, but if the previous years have
been well cared for, much may be left to habit,
and a wise governess will take care of any awk-
wardnesses incidental to girlhood.

We have now the child's hair to speak about.
The mode of wearing it hanging loose is much
the best for it ; but, we think, out of doors, it
should be tucked up or shaded by the hat or sun-
bonnet, as it will fade in the air and sunlight to
the colour of hay. It should never be cut. The
finest hair in the world grows on the heads of

Dutch and German women, who have never had scissors applied to it. If it is never cut, it will never want cutting under ordinary circumstances; but if it falls off, or is abnormally thin, *then* cut the ends every month. Neither should grease be used to a child's hair: it does not need it. It should be washed daily with soft water, and, when dry, well brushed. This is all the care necessary for rapid and ample growth.

The eyes should not be suffered to be tried by reading at twilight or candlelight, and *plenty* of sleep should be given before midnight ; girls should go to bed at seven till they are twelve years old, and rise early.

In nothing is it of more importance to take time by the forelock than in the matter of beauty. Care of it in childhood never loses its ultimate reward, and spares much future trouble.

We commend the subject to the more serious consideration of mothers.

THE END.

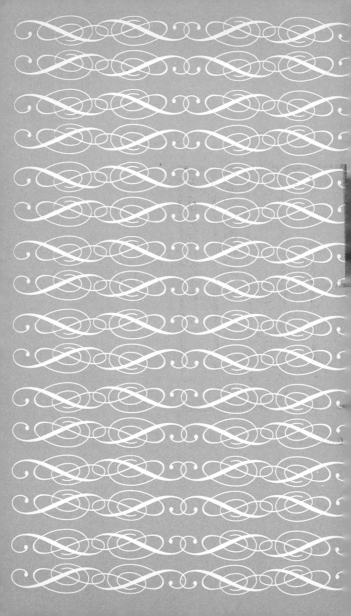